LUNG CANCER

UNDERSTANDING AND CAREFULLY
DEALING WITH LUNG CANCER

DR. A. RAMOS

Contents

INTRODUCTION 3

CHAPTER ONE 9

What Lung Cancer Means 9

Lung Composition and Operation 14

Anatomical Data..14

Protection of the immune system 18

Several types of lung cancer 19

Other Groups 21

Hazard Factors 24

CHAPTER TWO 28

Significance and Representations 30

Early screening and identification...............................35

Evaluating..40

CHAPTER THREE 46

Phase and Prediction 46

Limited versus Extensive Stages of Small Cell Lung Cancer (SCLC)
....48

Therapy Options..52

Palliative Health Care 58

Dietary support 64

CHAPTER FOUR 67

Adaptability and Follow-up 71

Prevention Techniques and Lifestyle Modifications 77

CHAPTER FIVE 84

Effects on the Emotional and Psychological Level 84

CONCLUSION 92

THE END 95

INTRODUCTION

Lung cancer represents one type of lung cancer that typically originates from the cells lining the airways. It is one of the most deadly and common forms of cancer worldwide. NSCLC and small cell lung cancer (SCLC) are the two main types of lung cancer that are frequently detected.

Lung cancer that is not small cell:

Non-small cell lung cancer (NSCLC) is classified into three subtypes: adenocarcinoma, squamous cell carcinoma, and giant cell carcinoma.

Non-small cell lung cancer accounts for about 85% of lung cancer cases (NSCLC).

Spread and Growth: Generally speaking, it expands more slowly than SCLC.

Lung cancer with small cells, or SCLC:

The defining feature of small-cell lung cancer (SCLC) is the rapid proliferation of tiny cancer cells, which often lead to large tumors.

Aggression: SCLC is generally more aggressive and has a higher propensity to spread to other parts of the body.

Pulmonary cancer risk factors include:

Cigarette smoking: Smoking is the main cause of lung cancer. Smoking significantly increases the risk of lung cancer, though nonsmokers can also get it.

Lung cancer risk has been associated with exposure to secondhand smoke.

Radon is a naturally occurring radioactive gas. Long-term exposure to it can be dangerous.

workplace Exposures: There is a possibility that lung cancer is caused by exposure to certain workplace hazards, including asbestos and diesel exhaust.

A family history of the disease may increase a person's risk of developing lung cancer.

Air Pollution: Exposure to high amounts of air pollution for an extended length of time may be dangerous.

The signs of lung cancer:

Common signs and symptoms of lung cancer include:

- Chronic cough
- A chest ache
- trouble breathing
- spitting out blood
- Weariness

Why am I getting thinner?

Assessing and Arranging:

Diagnostic imaging studies including biopsies and CT scans are commonly employed.

Therapy decisions are guided by the staging procedure, which aids in determining the extent of cancer progression.

Therapy Options:

Immunotherapy, targeted therapy, radiation, chemotherapy, surgery, or a combination of these are available as forms of treatment.

The treatment plan is determined by a number of criteria, including the patient's overall health and the type and stage of their lung cancer.

Expectation:

The prognosis is influenced by the kind of lung cancer, the stage of diagnosis, and the response to treatment.

Quick identification can improve outcomes significantly.

As a major public health concern, lung cancer highlights the importance of stopping smoking, early detection, and innovative treatment approaches to improve survival rates and quality of life.

CHAPTER ONE

What Lung Cancer Means

Lung cancer is a type of malignant tumor that arises from cells lining the airways in the lung tissues. The tumor's growth and obstruction of the lungs' normal function may have an effect on breathing and oxygen exchange. Worldwide, a considerable proportion of cancer-related deaths are caused by two main types of lung cancer: small cell lung cancer (SCLC) and non-small cell lung cancer (NSCLC).

Lung cancer that is not small cell:

This accounts for about 85% of cases of lung cancer.

include variants such as adenocarcinoma, squamous cell carcinoma, and large cell carcinoma etc.

is more likely than lung cancer with small cells to grow and spread slowly.

Lung cancer with small cells, or SCLC:

responsible for 15% of lung cancer cases.

This type of cancer is characterized by the rapid proliferation of small cancer cells that often result in large tumors.

Notorious for its early inclination to spread and for being ferocious.

Risky Components:

Smoking: As the main cause of lung cancer, smoking has a direct correlation with the disease's progression.

Secondhand Smoke: There is a greater risk when you are close to someone who has been smoking.

Examples of occupational exposures include exposure to asbestos, radon, and certain workplace hazards.

Family History: If a member of your family has had lung cancer, your risk may be higher.

Air pollution is the result of extended exposure to excessive air pollution levels.

Symptoms:

Lung cancer frequently manifests as chest pain, shortness of breath, blood in the cough, tiredness, and unexplained weight loss.

Assessing and Arranging:

Often, a sample is required to confirm the diagnosis, which is determined by imaging tests (CT and PET scans).

Therapy decisions are influenced by the stage of cancer spread.

Therapy Options:

Surgery, radiation therapy, chemotherapy, targeted therapy, and immunotherapy are some of the potential treatment options.

The treatment plan is determined by a number of criteria, including the patient's overall health and the type and stage of their lung cancer.

Expectation:

The prognosis is influenced by the kind of lung cancer, the stage of diagnosis, and the response to treatment.

Screenings can significantly improve outcomes by identifying issues early.

Lung cancer is a serious public health concern with the goal of improving patient outcomes. It is critical to prioritize prevention, early detection, and innovative treatment approaches.

The lungs, which are vital parts of the respiratory system, perform the exchange of oxygen and carbon dioxide, which enables the body to breathe and support many physiological functions. The following is a summary of the anatomy and functions of the lungs:

Anatomical Data

The bronchi and cholera:

The windpipe, or trachea, is the tube that carries air from the mouth and nose to the lungs.

The trachea divided into two bronchi, each of which led to a single lung.

Bronchioles:

The bronchi further divide into microscopic passageways called bronchioles inside the lungs.

The alveoli

Bronchioles terminate in tiny air sacs known as alveoli.

Alveoli, which are surrounded by blood vessels, are where gas exchange occurs.

The Lobes and Their Lobules:

The right lung has three lobes (upper, middle, and lower), and the left lung has two lobes (upper and lower).

Lobes are further broken into the smaller components called lobules.

Multiple:

The lungs are enclosed by the pleura, a double-layered membrane.

The pleura reduces the amount of friction that happens between the chest wall and the lungs when breathing.

Position:

Take a breath (ventilate):

The two primary functions of the lungs are breathing and ventilation.

During inhalation, or breathing, the diaphragm contracts and the rib cage expands, creating a negative pressure that draws air into the lungs.

During expiration, air is expelled out of the lungs as the diaphragm relaxes and the ribcage contracts.

Transform of Gas:

Red blood cell hemoglobin is bound by inhaled air oxygen as it diffuses into the bloodstream through the alveoli.

Carbon dioxide waste product diffuses into the alveoli for expiration at the same time as blood.

Oxygen Transport:

Rich in oxygen, blood is pushed from the lungs into the left atrium of the heart into the body's circulation, where it supplies nutrients to the tissues and organs.

The Removal of Carbon Dioxide:

The carbon dioxide produced during cellular metabolism is transported back to the lungs through the circulation.

When it is expelled during breathing, the respiratory cycle is considered complete.

Control of pH:

An essential part of maintaining the body's acid-base equilibrium is blood carbon dioxide regulation, which is carried out by the lungs.

Protection of the immune system

The respiratory system's mucous membranes and microscopic hair-like structures called cilia help to remove and trap bacteria, viruses, and other particles, bolstering the body's defenses against them.

Understanding the structure and function of the lungs is essential to appreciating their importance in respiratory physiology and overall health. Healthy lung function is essential for sustaining life and a variety of bodily processes.

Several types of lung cancer

Lung cancer can be classified into two basic types based on the microscopic features of the cancer cells: small cell lung cancer (SCLC) and non-small cell lung cancer (NSCLC). Each category has a variety of variants, and selecting an appropriate course of treatment requires an understanding of these variations. The main types of lung cancer are as follows:

Lung cancer that is not small cell:

adenocarcinomas:

This subtype of NSCLC is the most frequent and is typically observed in the outer region of the lungs.

appears frequently in both nonsmokers and former smokers.

expands normally more slowly than other subtypes.

Squamous cell carcinoma:

situated in the middle section of the lungs, frequently adjacent to a bronchus.

usually associated with a history of smoking.

maybe connected to particular precancerous changes in the lung.

An enormous cancer cell:

a subtype of NSCLC less common.

Cells appear distorted and large under a microscope.

occurs along the entire length of the lung.

Other Groups

Among the subtypes of NSCLC, sarcoid and adenosquamous carcinomas are two less common versions.

Lung cancer with small cells, or SCLC:

Small-cell carcinoma:

responsible for 15% of lung cancer cases.

composed of small cells that divide quickly and have a tendency to spread swiftly.

usually associated with a history of smoking.

responds well to early chemotherapy in most cases, although it often comes back.

Combined or Combination Types:

There are also cases where lung cancers have characteristics from both NSCLC and SCLC. These are called blended or mixed types.

Lung Cancer That Is Not Specific:

Some lung tumors may end up classified as undefinable since they do not neatly fit into any of the established categories.

The distinctions between NSCLC and SCLC impact treatment decisions since the two types respond differently to various therapies. In addition, the characteristics of the tumor itself, the patient's overall health, and the stage of the disease may all play a role in treatment decisions.

Making the right treatment decision for someone with lung cancer is aided by an accurate diagnosis that considers results from both molecular testing and histological evaluation. Scientific advances that continue to uncover new details about the molecular and genetic makeup of lung cancer are leading to the development of more targeted and customized therapeutic approaches.

Hazard Factors

Lung cancer risk factors are associated with many risk variables. Notably, even while these traits may raise the risk, lung cancer does not always occur in individuals who possess them; in fact, some people may not have any risk factors at all and yet develop the disease. Typical lung cancer risk factors include the following:

Usage of tobacco:

Primary Risk Factor: Smoking cigarettes is the main cause of lung cancer. It is the main factor in cases of lung cancer.

Being in the vicinity of secondhand smoke, often known as passive smoking, increases the risk as well, particularly for people who do not smoke.

Exposure to Radiation Gas:

Organic Gas: Extended exposure to high radon concentrations can be extremely dangerous. Radon is a colorless, odorless radioactive gas that can infiltrate through walls and into dwellings.

Hazards at Work:

Asbestos: Workplace exposure to asbestos, a substance used in building and insulation, has been linked to an increased risk of lung cancer.

Other Carcinogens: If you are exposed to certain carcinogens at work, such diesel exhaust, arsenic, chromium, or nickel, your risk of developing cancer may rise.

The Family's Past:

Due to possible genetic vulnerability or common environmental exposures, a family history of lung cancer may raise an individual's risk.

The individual's history of lung cancer:

Lung cancer recurrence is more common in people with a history of the disease.

Respiratory conditions

Patients with persistent lung ailments, especially those with chronic obstructive pulmonary disease (COPD), have an increased chance of developing lung cancer.

Pulmonary fibrosis may be more likely in cases of lung tissue scarring.

Prior Radiation Therapy:

Lung cancer risk may be higher in individuals who have undergone radiation therapy to the chest, regardless of whether it was for another type of cancer.

Air contamination

The risk may rise with prolonged exposure to elevated air pollution levels, such as those caused by particulate matter and certain pollutants.

CHAPTER TWO

Dietary Components:

Diet has a complex impact on the risk of lung cancer. Consuming a diet low in fruits and vegetables may put you at risk, according to some research.

Genetic Variables:

Hereditary genetic changes may lead to an elevated risk of lung cancer, despite the fact that these circumstances are comparatively uncommon.

Human Infection with Papillomavirus (HPV):

Though it is most well-known for its association with cervical cancer, HPV infection has also been linked to an elevated risk of lung cancer.

Individuals with established risk factors, particularly those with a history of smoking, ought to undergo routine testing and maintain close communication with their medical providers. Screenings for lung cancer early on can significantly improve outcomes for those who have a high risk of developing the disease. Furthermore, living a healthy lifestyle that includes avoiding environmental pollutants and quitting smoking may help reduce the risk of lung cancer.

There can be variations in the signs and symptoms of lung cancer depending on the kind, stage, and degree of the disease's invasion into nearby tissues. Some patients with early-stage lung cancer may not even exhibit any symptoms. The following are typical signs and symptoms:

Coughing nonstop:

The most common symptom of lung cancer is a chronic cough that either never goes away or becomes worse with time.

Loss of Blood:

Hemateptysis—the discharge of blood or bloody sputum—may occur in extremely uncommon cases.

Trouble breathing:

The impact of the tumor on lung function may result in dyspnea or difficulty breathing.

Chest Pain:

The tumor's pressure on surrounding nerves or the chest wall may result in sudden, mild, or chronic chest pain.

Gasping for air

Wheezing or a persistent raspy sound may be the result of breathing difficulties, especially if the tumor obstructs the airways.

Hoarseness sound:

voice irregularities, including hoarseness, may arise if the tumor destroys the nerves that control the voice chords.

Unexpected Loss of Weight:

Lung cancer is among the numerous cancers that can result in inadvertent weight loss, often rather significant.

Fatigue:

Weakness and fatigue may be long-lasting effects of lung cancer, particularly as the disease progresses.

Diminished Appetite:

A decrease in appetite and a shift in eating patterns are possible.

More than one respiratory infection:

Recurrent infections such as pneumonia or bronchitis might result from immune system weakness caused by lung cancer.

Face and neck swelling:

The neck and face may swell as a result of a lung tumor that affects the lymph nodes or blood vessels.

Bone pain:

Lung cancer that has spread to the bones can cause bone discomfort, generally in the hips or back.

Head Pain:

Metastases in the brain can cause headaches, seizures, or other neurological disorders.

Pain in the Joints:

One possible cause of joint pain is metastasis from cancer.

It's important to remember that many lung cancer symptoms could just as easily be caused by other illnesses. However, if you experience new symptoms or if your condition worsens, you should see a physician, especially if you have a known lung cancer risk factor. Early detection and diagnosis are critical to improving treatment outcomes. If you or someone you know is exhibiting concerning symptoms, it's imperative that you get medical attention straight once.

Early screening and identification

Early detection and screening are crucial for improving the prognosis of people who have a high risk of lung cancer. Finding lung cancer early on, when it is more treatable, usually before symptoms manifest, is the aim of screening. The following crucial elements are involved in lung cancer screening and early detection:

1. Categories at High Risk:

Age and Smoking History: It is typically recommended that those between the ages of 50 and 80 who have a significant smoking history that is, a history of smoking one pack of cigarettes per day for twenty years get a lung cancer screening.

Former Smokers: Individuals who stopped smoking within the last 15 years may still be considered to be at high risk.

2. The term "low-dose computed tomography" (LDCT):

Low-dose CT scanning is the method that is advised for the detection of lung cancer (LDCT).

Advantages: LDCT may provide more effective treatment by identifying small lung nodules and early-stage lung cancers.

3. Screening Frequency:

Annual Screening: For high-risk individuals, LDCT scans are typically recommended annually.

4. Together, we decide on:

Consult with your healthcare provider: Anyone considering a lung cancer screening should consult with their healthcare provider to weigh the advantages and risks.

Efficient Decision-Making: Participant awareness of the potential benefits of early identification as well as the risks, such as overdiagnosis and false positives, is ensured by collaborative decision-making.

5. Early Recognition and Handling:

More therapy Options: Getting lung cancer detected early improves the prognosis and opens up more options for therapy.

Surgical Procedures: Lobectomies or wedge resections are two possible surgical procedures for treating early-stage lung cancer.

6. Follow-Up on Lung Nodules:

Follow-Up Imaging: If lung nodules are seen but do not immediately seem to be malignant, doctors may suggest doing more imaging to monitor any changes over time.

7. Upcoming Research and Advancements:

Ongoing Research: This research aims to enhance overall outcomes, develop more precise screening methods for lung cancer, and develop early detection approaches.

Emerging Technologies: Scientific and technology advancements may lead to the creation of new screening techniques and tools.

8. Public health initiatives:

Public health efforts and awareness campaigns aim to educate the public about the importance of screening for lung cancer, especially for individuals who are at high risk.

Those who have a high risk of lung cancer should discuss their screening options with their medical providers. Screening for early detection can significantly improve the chances of a successful course of therapy and long-term survival. Furthermore, living a healthy lifestyle that includes avoiding environmental pollutants and quitting smoking may help reduce the risk of lung cancer.

Evaluating

The diagnosis of lung cancer requires a comprehensive evaluation that includes a physical examination, imaging studies, a medical history, and often a biopsy to confirm the presence of malignant cells. The following are the crucial steps in identifying lung cancer:

1. medical history and physical examination:

An authorized healthcare provider documents the patient's symptoms, overall health, and lung cancer risk factors.

During a thorough physical examination, the chest and respiratory system are the primary emphasis regions.

2. Exams for imaging:

The initial imaging test for abnormalities in the lungs is a chest X-ray.

The Computed Tomography (CT) scan makes it simpler to detect and identify tumors and nodules by providing detailed cross-sectional images of the lungs.

By measuring the amount of metabolic activity in the lungs, a PET scan can reveal information about the cancer's spread.

3. Sputum Cytology:

With a microscope, sputum is examined to search for malignant cells.

4. A postmortem

The most reliable method for determining the kind and existence of cancer is a biopsy.

Needle Biopsy: A thin, hollow needle is used to extract lung tissue for examination.

Bronchoscopy: A flexible tube fitted with a light and camera is placed into the airways to collect samples of lung tissue.

Thoracentesis: If there is fluid surrounding the lungs, or pleural effusion, a sample of the fluid may be drawn for analysis.

Surgical Biopsy: Under some conditions, a surgical procedure may be necessary in order to collect a larger tissue sample.

5. Testing in a lab:

The genetic and molecular characteristics of the cancer cells are investigated using molecular testing.

identifies specific DNA alterations or mutations that may affect treatment decisions.

Determining one's eligibility for targeted therapy is especially crucial when dealing with non-small cell lung cancer (NSCLC).

6. Getting Ready:

After the diagnosis is confirmed, staging determines the extent of cancer spread.

The TNM System determines the stage (I to IV) based on the tumor's size, involvement of lymph nodes, and metastasis.

7. Examinations for Heart Function:

Assesses lung function to determine how well the lungs are functioning.

8. Speaking with the interdisciplinary group:

A multidisciplinary team of oncologists, pulmonologists, radiologists, and pathologists collaborates to develop a personalized therapy plan.

9. The Second Opinion:

Obtaining a second opinion is recommended in difficult cases to ensure a thorough and accurate diagnosis.

A correct diagnosis is necessary to develop an effective treatment strategy that is tailored to the type and stage of lung cancer. Early diagnosis allows for timely intervention and improved treatment outcomes. When undergoing diagnostic testing, patients should actively participate in discussions with their healthcare providers and ask questions on any element of their diagnosis and suggested treatment plan.

CHAPTER THREE

Phase and Prediction

Staging and prognosis are important concepts to grasp in order to estimate the extent of lung cancer and predict its likely course. Staging includes evaluating the tumor's size, spread to neighboring lymph nodes, and possibility of organ metastases. The prognosis is an estimation of what is anticipated based on several factors. Here's an outline of it:

1. The Course of Lung Cancer:

TNM staging method: This approach is commonly used in the treatment of lung cancer. Three key points are taken into account:

T (Tumor): Specifies the size of the main tumor.

The letter N (Node) indicates that lymph nodes nearby are affected.

The letter M (metastasis) denotes the presence of malignancy that has spread to distant organs.

Stages:

Stage 0: Carcinoma in situ, in which there is cancer but the abnormal cells have not metastasized to nearby organs.

Stages I and II: In the early stages of lung cancer, these are localized tumors that have not spread much to nearby structures.

Stages IIIA and IIIB: Wider involvement of neighboring structures or lymph nodes as a result of locally advanced cancer.

Stage IV: Cancer that has spread to other organs and is extremely metastatic.

Limited versus Extensive Stages of Small Cell Lung Cancer (SCLC)

Limited stage SCLC is confined to one side of the chest, whereas extensive stage extends beyond one side. These two stages are sometimes distinguished from one another.

2. Forecasting variables:

Histology: Based on the type of lung cancer (small cell lung cancer, SCLC vs. non-small cell lung cancer, NSCLC), the prognosis varies for each.

Greater tumor size may indicate a more advanced stage of the disease and a less favorable prognosis.

Lymph Node Involvement: The prognosis is largely influenced by how well the malignancy can spread to nearby lymph nodes.

Metastasis: A far-off metastasis significantly affects the prognosis.

Performance Status: The patient's ability to accept and respond to treatment is influenced by their overall health and functional state.

Genetic Mutations: Some genetic mutations might influence the prognosis and how the body reacts to particular treatments.

3. Consequences of Treatment:

Treatment Options: The stage of a cancer dictates the course of care; advanced-stage malignancies may require a combination of radiation, chemotherapy, surgery, targeted therapy, or immunotherapy, whereas early-stage cancers are usually operated on.

Treatment objectives can be curative (for diseases in their early stages) or palliative (to control symptoms and improve quality of life).

4. Survival Ratios:

Five-Year Survival Rates: Based on the kind and stage of lung cancer, survival rates vary. The five-year survival rate for malignancies in their early stages is often higher than that of cancers in their advanced stages.

5. Individual Variation:

Each patient's response to treatment may differ significantly from the prognosis, which is merely an estimate.

Therapy Advancements: Current research and novel approaches to therapy continue to impact prognosis and outcomes.

To develop a personalized treatment plan and set realistic expectations for patients and their families, it is critical to understand the stage and prognosis of lung cancer. Regular follow-up and communication with the medical team are essential during the course of treatment.

Therapy Options

Depending on the type of lung cancer, the stage at which it has progressed, the overall health of the patient, and other individual factors, different lung cancer treatments are prescribed. Treatments for lung cancer typically include immunotherapy, chemotherapy, radiation therapy, targeted therapy, supportive care, and surgery. In the multimodal therapy technique, these strategies are often employed in conjunction. The primary therapeutic modalities are outlined below:

1. Surgical:

A lobectomy is the whole excision of the lung lobe containing the tumor.

Removal of a smaller portion of the lung, known as a wedge resection or segmentectomy, is appropriate in some situations, especially when maintaining lung function is crucial.

When the primary bronchus is affected by the cancer, a pneumonectomy a complete removal of the lung is typically performed.

2. Chemotherapy therapy:

Chemotherapy is a systemic treatment that goes after quickly dividing cancer cells all over the body, killing them.

Combination therapy: when given in conjunction with other medications, it is utilized to boost efficacy.

Adjuvant or Neoadjuvant: Applied prior to or following surgery in either case to minimize tumor size or prevent recurrence.

3. Radiation therapy by X-ray:

External Beam Radiation: Powerful beams are aimed at malignant cells and destroy them. It can serve as the primary course of treatment, be taken on its own, in combination with chemotherapy or surgery, or neither.

Stereotactic body radiation therapy, or SBRT: Targeted high-dose radiation that is accurate and beneficial for some early-stage lung malignancies.

Radiation therapy can be used as a palliative approach in cases when symptoms are advanced, or as an adjuvant intervention following surgery.

4. Focused Intervention:

Some molecular targets, such as alterations or mutations in cancer cells, are the focus of targeted treatment drugs.

Certain genetic abnormalities identified in non-small cell lung cancer (NSCLC) can be targeted with medicines such as ALK, ROS1, and EGFR inhibitors.

5. The immune system:

Checkpoint Inhibitors: Immunotherapy drugs such as PD-1 and PD-L1 inhibitors bolster the body's defenses against malignant cells.

often used for advanced non-small cell lung cancer, especially when PD-L1 expression is elevated.

6. Offering Assistive Healthcare:

Palliative care: Helps patients with lung cancer that is advanced or incurable to manage their symptoms, lessen their discomfort, and improve their quality of life.

Nutritional Support: It's important to receive enough nutrients for overall health and healing.

7. Clinical Examinations:

Investigative Therapies: Participating in clinical trials may provide you access to novel medicines or novel combinations of drugs that are already on the market.

8. Personalized Medical Attention:

Molecular profiling involves detecting specific genetic alterations or abnormalities present in the tumor to help guide therapy decisions.

The individualized approach involves creating a treatment plan based on the specific type and characteristics of the patient's cancer.

9. Following Program Care:

Regular check-ins and imaging are essential parts of follow-up care, as is keeping an eye out for any signs of recurrence or treatment-related adverse effects.

The kind and stage of the lung cancer, the presence of specific genetic abnormalities, and the patient's overall condition all affect the therapy decision. A multidisciplinary team of medical professionals develops a personalized treatment plan for each patient. Advances in lung cancer research and treatment choices continue to impact the landscape of lung cancer care, with a focus on improving outcomes and quality of life.

Palliative Health Care

The aim of comprehensive lung cancer treatment is to improve the quality of life for patients with advanced or terminal lung cancer, and palliative care is an essential component of this approach. Cancer treatment strategies incorporate palliative care at every stage to address the physical, emotional, and psychosocial needs of patients. It is not limited to use in last-mile circumstances. A synopsis of palliative treatment for lung cancer is as follows:

1. The Division of Palliative Care:

Multidisciplinary Approach: Members of a palliative care team frequently include specialists, nurses, social workers, and doctors with expertise in palliative care.

2. Handling Symptoms:

Palliative care successfully treats cancer-related pain by using medications, treatments, and other strategies.

Managing symptoms such as fatigue, nausea, dyspnea, and other physical aches and pains in order to enhance the patient's overall health.

3. Support for Psychosocial Problems and Emotions:

Therapy and Counseling: Providing emotional support through support groups, therapy, and counseling to patients and their families.

In managing the psychological aftermath of a lung cancer diagnosis and how it impacts day-to-day functioning, anxiety and depression are addressed.

4. Communication and Decision-Making:

The patient's prognosis, potential treatments, and goals for their care should all be openly and honestly communicated.

Advance care planning refers to assisting with discussions regarding living wills, advance directives, and end-of-life desires.

5. Support for Existentialism and Spirituality:

Spiritual care is attending to the spiritual needs of a patient and helping their family members who are looking for a sense of purpose, meaning, or community.

6. Final Days of Life Care:

Comfort measures: Taking action to make sure that the patient's last comfort and dignity come first.

Hospice Care: During the final stages of a disease, focusing on comfort and quality of life, this approach is taken when appropriate.

7. A comprehensive plan

The term "holistic needs assessment" refers to the process of evaluating a person's physical, emotional, social, and spiritual needs.

Family members and caregivers should be supported by providing aid to those who are essential to the patient's care.

8. Organizing oncology care in coordination:

Integrated Care: Palliative care is a holistic approach to treatment that is often provided in conjunction with therapies aimed at curing or prolonging life.

9. Information & Knowledge:

Education of the Patient and Family: Providing information about the disease, possible therapies, and managing expectations.

One of the main facets of empowerment is the ability of the patient and family to make decisions about their own care.

10. Assistance in Grieving:

Grief counseling: Helping and advising family members following a patient's death.

creating connections between families and community resources to offer additional support.

Palliative care is an integral part of the healthcare system because it provides comfort and support to patients throughout the course of their lung cancer journey. Prioritizing the patient, the strategy tailors care to each individual's specific needs and preferences. The goal is to enhance overall quality of life for lung cancer patients and their families.

Dietary support

Because the illness and its treatments may alter a patient's appetite, weight, and overall nutritional status, patients with lung cancer need to receive nutritional care. Eating healthily contributes to overall welfare, energy maintenance, and the body's ability to cope with the negative effects of cancer treatment. Lung cancer patients should consider the following crucial elements when receiving nutritional support:

1. Customized Food Programs:

Speak with a Registered Dietitian or Nutritionist; they can ascertain a person's nutritional needs and provide a personalized diet plan.

Dietary preferences and Difficulties Should Be Taken into Account: The plan should take the patient's food preferences, eating challenges, and other behaviors into consideration.

2. Maintaining an Adequate Energy Consumption:

Requirements for Energy: People with lung cancer must meet their needs for energy, or calories, in order to maintain strength and support body functions.

Meals That Are Small and Frequent: Eating smaller, more frequent meals throughout the day may be more tolerable for those who are suffering from hunger swings.

3. Consumption of proteins:

Protein: To sustain muscle growth and repair, an adequate diet is necessary.

Protein-rich foods that ought to be a part of a diet include beans, nuts, dairy products, fish, poultry, and lean meats.

4. Changing with the Appetite:

There are situations in which doctors may provide appetite enhancers to increase food intake.

Flavor Enhancements: Food can have its flavor enhanced by adding herbs, spices, and flavor enhancers.

5. Appropriate Hydration

Hydration: Keeping enough water on hand is essential for overall health and for cancer therapy in particular.

Eating foods high in water content, like soups, fruits, and vegetables, is advised.

6. Nutrient-Rich Foods:

Increasing Nutrient Intake: Give foods that are rich in nutrients and an excellent source of vitamins and minerals priority.

Colorful Fruits and Vegetables, Whole Grains: Consume whole grains along with colorful fruits and vegetables to gain a variety of nutrients.

7. Handling Intestinal Issues:

Handling Nausea and Vomiting: If nausea is a problem, work with medical experts to manage symptoms and identify foods that are tolerated.

Fiber Intake: Varying based on Digestive Comfort; during therapy, a low-fiber diet may be beneficial for certain people.

8. Additional Foods:

Meal replacement shakes or nutritional supplements could be recommended in the event that oral intake is insufficient.

Vitamin and mineral supplements: Use supplements when necessary to address specific dietary deficiencies.

9. Observe and modify as necessary:

Regularly observing the diet plan, adjusting as needed, and assessing nutritional status are all part of frequent monitoring.

It is important to keep lines of communication open with the medical team about any changes in appetite, weight, or nutritional concerns.

10. Support for Reducing Weight:

Maintenance of a Healthy Weight: For those who have inadvertently lost weight, the food plan may include strategies for increasing or maintaining weight.

11. Assistance with feelings:

Addressing Emotional Problems: Psychotherapy and emotional support for individuals experiencing emotional problems related to shifts in body mass, appetite, or eating habits.

A patient with lung cancer should work closely with the medical team to develop and adjust a nutrition plan that suits their individual needs, with the assistance of a qualified dietitian. The goals are to promote the body's tolerance to treatment, optimize nutritional intake, and improve overall well-being during the cancer journey.

Adaptability and Follow-up

With regard to lung cancer, the term "survivor" refers to the period of time that elapses following the conclusion of active therapy. People monitor their health throughout this phase, manage any adverse effects from treatment, and attend to their physical and emotional needs. The following are essential components of follow-up care and survivability in lung cancer:

1. Scheme for Survivorship Care:

Tailored Approach: A survivor's care plan include details about their medical background, therapies they received, and recommendations for additional care.

Assistive Care: A personalized survivorship care plan is created by the medical team, which consists of additional experts and oncologists.

2. Behavioural Visits:

Regular Monitoring: During follow-up appointments with the medical staff, the patient's overall health is regularly assessed, and any potential adverse effects of therapy are discussed.

Consultation Frequency: The number of follow-up visits may vary depending on the kind and stage of lung cancer, the therapy being administered, and the patient's health.

3. Diagnostic and imaging examinations:

Regular Imaging: To check for any signs of recurrence, imaging exams such as CT scans and chest X-rays are frequently performed.

Pulmonary Function Tests: These tests are used to assess lung function, particularly in patients who have had lung surgery.

4. Keeping an eye out for any fallout later:

Cardiopulmonary Health: Keeping an eye out for any potential long-term consequences on the heart and lungs, especially if radiation therapy was recommended as a recommended course of treatment.

Assessment of Bone Health: Identification of potential issues with particular therapies.

5. General Health and Lifestyle:

It is advised to lead a healthy lifestyle that includes giving up smoking, eating a balanced diet, and engaging in frequent exercise.

Emotional support is defined as promoting mental well-being and providing resources to help cope with the psychological fallout from having cancer.

6. Managing Prolonged Negative Impacts:

Handling Side Effects: Extended treatment side effects, such weariness, neuropathy, or irregularities in cognition, will still be handled and managed.

Rehabilitation Services: If required, utilizing rehabilitation services to address any functional difficulties resulting from treatment.

7. Resources & Programs for Survivorship:

One approach to locate supportive programs is to take part in survivorship initiatives that offer information, assistance, and resources to individuals following treatment.

Community Resources: establishing ties with local resources and support networks to receive ongoing help.

8. Watch out for tumors that metastasize:

Cancer surveillance is keeping an eye out for the formation of second primary tumors, especially when the patient has a history of smoking or other risk factors.

9. Together, we decide on:

Encouraging active participation in the decision-making process for follow-up care and attending to any concerns or questions raised.

10. Making Advance Care Ready:

Talks about Advance Care Planning: We'll keep talking about advance care planning, including decisions about future medical procedures and preferences for end-of-life care.

Survivorship care is centered around helping patients transition from active treatment to a phase of ongoing monitoring and support. The goals are to promote overall wellbeing, manage any treatment-related side effects, and optimize health. Lung cancer survivability requires a whole-person approach to health, adherence to follow-up care plans, and honest dialogue with the medical staff.

Prevention Techniques and Lifestyle Modifications

By implementing specific lifestyle modifications and preventative measures, the risk of lung cancer can be considerably reduced. A healthy lifestyle can help lower overall risk even though an individual may not be able to control certain risk factors such as genetic predisposition and environmental exposures. Important lifestyle and preventive actions for lung cancer include the following:

1. Giving Up The Smoke:

The most frequent cause of lung cancer is smoking, which is the primary risk factor. Giving up smoking is the best way to lower risk.

Support in Quitting: To effectively quit smoking, seek out medical professionals' advice, counseling, and programs specifically designed to assist individuals in quitting.

2. Stopping Smoke Exposure

Reduce Exposure: Steer clear of secondhand smoke at all costs as it increases the risk of lung cancer.

3. How to Combat Radon Gas:

Testing and Mitigation: Look for naturally occurring radioactive gas radon in homes, as it can seep into buildings. Should higher levels of exposure be discovered, take steps to mitigate and lower exposure.

4. Safety at Work:

Protective Measures: Workers who perform jobs that expose them to asbestos, diesel exhaust, chemicals, or other carcinogens should follow the recommended safety procedures.

5. Environmental Knowledge:

Air Quality: Take the necessary precautions and be aware of environmental carcinogens and air pollutants to lessen your exposure to them.

Workplace Safety: Follow safety procedures when working with materials that may expose you to hazardous materials.

6. A wholesome diet

Maintain a well-balanced body by eating a diet rich in fruits, vegetables, whole grains, lean proteins, and other nutrients.

To protect your cells from damage, eat a diet high in foods high in antioxidants.

7. Regular Workout:

Exercise: Regular exercise has been associated with a decreased risk of lung cancer, so it is advised that you engage in it.

Keep a Healthy Weight: Try to avoid obesity and keep a healthy weight to lower your chance.

8. Cut Back on Alcohol Consumption:

Moderate Consumption: If you do drink, do so in moderation. Excessive alcohol consumption is associated with an increased risk of developing certain forms of cancer.

9. Monitoring for the presence of lung cancer:

Individuals at High Risk: If you or a loved one has a high risk of developing lung cancer, such as heavy smoking in the past or present, speak with medical professionals about getting screened for the disease.

10. Genetic counseling:

Family History: To find out their genetic risk, people with a family history of lung cancer may find that genetic counseling is a useful option.

11. Defense against the Sun:

Skin Protection: To reduce your risk of developing skin cancer, which can occasionally spread to your lungs, protect your skin from harmful UV rays.

12. vaccine

Vaccinations against influenza and pneumonia: Vaccinating against influenza and pneumonia in particular can help with preventative health.

13. Typical Health Exams:

Health Monitoring: Schedule routine examinations and screenings to detect and address potential health issues early on.

14. Ethical Lifestyle:

To manage your stress, engage in stress-relieving activities like mindfulness, yoga, or meditation.

Maintaining a healthy lifestyle and taking proactive preventative measures can significantly lower the risk of lung cancer. Prioritizing their overall health, being aware of their risk factors, and making informed decisions are all important. Adhering to suggested screening procedures and keeping in regular communication with medical professionals are further components of preventive care.

CHAPTER FIVE

Effects on the Emotional and Psychological Level

The patient, their loved ones, and caregivers may experience profound emotional and psychological effects following a lung cancer diagnosis. Coping with the psychological aspects of the journey and managing a range of emotions are crucial components of overcoming the obstacles that come with being diagnosed with lung cancer. The impact of lung cancer on an individual's emotions and mental state includes the following significant factors:

1. First Sensational Responses:

Shock and Denial: Many people experience shock before making an effort to refute the validity of their diagnosis.

Concerns about what lies ahead, how to manage the illness, and how it will impact day-to-day living can arise after receiving a lung cancer diagnosis.

2. Volcano of psychology:

Emotional Shifts: Coping with lung cancer can evoke a spectrum of feelings, including highs and lows, as well as periods of courage, optimism, and hope as well as dejection, fury, or fear.

3. Influence on the Psychology

Anxiety and Depression: For some people who show signs of anxiety or depression, support and intervention may be required.

Psychological Distress: There are a number of factors that can contribute to psychological distress, including uncertainty about the disease, difficulties related to treatment, and the impact on quality of life.

4. Innovative Methods:

Coping Mechanisms: People devise a range of coping mechanisms to handle the emotional burden. Asking for help from loved ones, engaging in activities they enjoy, and putting the present moment first are a few of these.

Support Groups: Joining a support group or counseling session can provide you with a forum for discussing your emotions and establishing relationships with others experiencing comparable circumstances.

5. Connection-Releasing Impact:

Family dynamics can be affected by a lung cancer diagnosis in a number of ways, including roles and responsibilities shifting, communication problems, and caregiving obligations.

Families must navigate the emotional terrain together, which requires open and honest communication.

6. dread of being socially unacceptable

Managing Stigma: People who have lung cancer may encounter stigma since the illness is frequently linked to smoking. Confronting and challenging misconceptions is essential, as is cultivating empathy.

7. Spirituality and existence-related worries:

Questions about Meaning: In an attempt to find purpose and direction in their lives, some people who have been diagnosed with cancer turn to existential and spiritual concerns.

Spiritual Support: Seeking pastoral care or counseling in order to receive existential or spiritual support can be beneficial.

8. Effects on One's Own Image

Physical Changes: Hair loss or weight fluctuations brought on by a treatment may impact a patient's self-worth and feelings about their bodies.

Self-Acceptance: Promoting self-acceptance and teaching people how to adapt to change are essential elements of mental wellness.

9. Challenges to Surviving:

Fear of Recurrence: It can be emotionally draining to constantly worry that, once cancer treatment is over, the fear will return.

Managing Survivability: Managing survival comprises finding a solution to enduring emotional problems and acclimating to a "new normal."

10. Connecting with medical professionals:

Keep Lines of Communication Open: Maintaining open lines of communication with healthcare professionals regarding emotional and psychological issues is crucial for comprehensive care.

Integrated Care: It is imperative that mental health services be a part of the comprehensive cancer care plan.

11. Hospice and Post-Memorial Support:

Complete Support: Palliative care provides complete support by addressing not only physical symptoms but also psychological and emotional issues.

12. Effects of Time on Life Quality:

The overall quality of life of an individual with lung cancer is significantly impacted by their emotional and psychological well-being.

Taking a comprehensive approach that recognizes the links between social, emotional, and physical health is required to address the psychological and emotional impacts of lung cancer. Seeking help from healthcare providers, mental health specialists, support groups, and immediate family members can help to promote a more resilient and adaptive coping process. Regular communication and a tailored approach to emotional care are essential components of a comprehensive lung cancer support system.

Lung cancer is an illness that is challenging and complex, impacting the patient as well as those close to them. From the disease's many forms and risk factors to the stages of diagnosis, available treatments, and survivor considerations, overcoming lung cancer entails overcoming a plethora of physical, psychological, and emotional obstacles.

By taking preventive measures, such as giving up smoking, being environmentally conscious, and maintaining a healthy lifestyle, the risk of lung cancer can be considerably reduced. Early detection through screening and prompt medical attention can improve treatment outcomes. The growing array of treatment options—which includes immunotherapy, surgery, chemotherapy, targeted therapy, and palliative care highlights the significance of a customized and multidisciplinary approach to care.

The psychological and emotional effects of lung cancer are profound, making open communication, coping strategies, and support networks essential. Providing ongoing monitoring, managing side effects, and preserving general health are all part of survivorship.

As awareness and research grow, we can anticipate improved outcomes, early detection methods, and innovative treatments. Enhancing the quality of life and care during the lung cancer trajectory requires fostering a collaborative and compassionate approach among medical professionals, people affected by lung cancer, and their support systems.

THE END